# Do~In

## Exercises for the

## Meridian System

## Of the Body

Francine Milford

Photographs by Paul, Larry and Francine Milford

**Caution**

The techniques, ideas, and suggestions presented in this book are not intended as a substitute for proper medical advice. Any application of the techniques, ideas, and suggestions in this book is at the reader's sole discretion and risk.

Printed in the United States of America

# Table of Contents

## Dedication


**This book is dedicated to all the Shiatsu, Yoga, Qigong, and Tai Chi practitioners who share their knowledge and joy of the flow of energy in the body.**

# Introduction

DoIn is a form of self shiatsu, or self massage. This ancient technique was sometimes used as a prelude, or warm-up, to more vigorous martial art exercises including Qigong, Tai Chi and Tae Kwon Do.

When used separately, these simple to learn and easy to do exercises can be used by anyone, regardless of their physical level of health.

Daily use of DoIn exercises can help your body to maintain health and vitality throughout the day.

Are you too busy to complete all the exercises at one time? No problem. With DoIn, although it is best to complete the series of exercises at one time, it is not necessary. You can complete sections of the DoIn exercises throughout the day.

Whenever you have feelings of stress or anxiety during the day, take a quick DoIn exercise break and revitalize the systems of your body.

These exercises can be practiced in the comfort of your own home, at the office, or while waiting in line.

Take a DoIn break today, you and your body deserve it.

**Chapter One**

**Introduction to Do~In**

Do-In, (pronounced dough-in), is an ancient exercise practice
that was brought to the United States by Michio Kushi in the
1960s. But Do-In didn't start then, it has existed for centuries.

Do-In became a more formally structured system more than
10,000 years ago. In rediscovering the precepts of Do-In, Kushi
acknowledges his debt to an enlightening experience during
meditation, and to the wisdom found in texts and teachings from
around the world. These teachings had a common source,
Kushi believes, and the unifying thread is the need and the
means for humans to adapt to the natural world around them.

The Do-In exercises were developed over the centuries in
oriental religions such as Shintoism, Hinduism, Taoism, and
Buddhism. Even though the DoIn exercises themselves are
physical practices and their purpose is to produce physical
health; spiritual harmony with the Universe is the ultimate goal.

As a form of self shiatsu, these self-help techniques often
resemble yoga postures. The exercises are designed to
improve, maintain and develop your overall general physical,
mental, as well as, emotional health and well-being.

DoIn exercises may be practiced by anyone and at anytime.
Even children may learn the simple and easy to do sequence of
exercises. There is no special equipment needed.

These exercises will help to open up the energy channels of
your body. These energy channels, called **Meridians,** include
every organ, tissue, and system of your body.

Do-In exercises were designed to release any blockages, or stagnant energy within the systems of your body to facilitate the free flow energy, called **Qi**, within the body. By accomplishing this, circulation is improved. DoIn will help you to feel warm, invigorated and energized!

The set of exercises are recommended to be performed as a series. In this course, we will learn about the various components of the exercises which include their benefits to the body. Then, at the end of the book, we will put them all together as a series of exercise, or into an exercise routine.

While there is nothing wrong with doing any part of the series of exercises, it is most beneficial to do the whole set of sequences when performing Do-In.

Even though there is no set time of day to perform Do-In exercises, it is recommended to do the Do-In exercises first thing in the morning, upon rising, and then throughout the day as you need to.

**To perform the Do-In exercises, it is important to remember a few things**.

**(1)** Keep a natural posture and remain relaxed throughout the exercises. Keep your knees slightly bent.

**(2)** Breathe normally. Most people catch themselves holding their breath when doing exercises. So please remember to breathe in through your nose and exhale out of your mouth throughout this entire series of exercises.

**(3)** Focus. Try to keep your mind free from outside disturbances. Try to clear your mind from any thoughts and feelings to maintain an empty mind. Keep your mind focused on the exercises that you are doing and on how your body is feeling while you are doing these exercises. You should become aware of the effect that the Do-In exercises are having on your body.

**(4)** Do NOT do the Do-In exercises for the stomach and legs if you are pregnant.

**(5)** Do not get discouraged.

**Caution Note**: If you feel tired, dizzy, or are in pain - STOP IMMEDIATELY and consult with your doctor.

Consult with your Doctor before beginning this or any other exercise program.

Once you have done the series of Do-In exercises over and over again a few times, it will become quite easy and natural for you to do them without looking at diagrams, etc. You will become aware of the natural flow of energy and will be able to work with them.

# To Begin

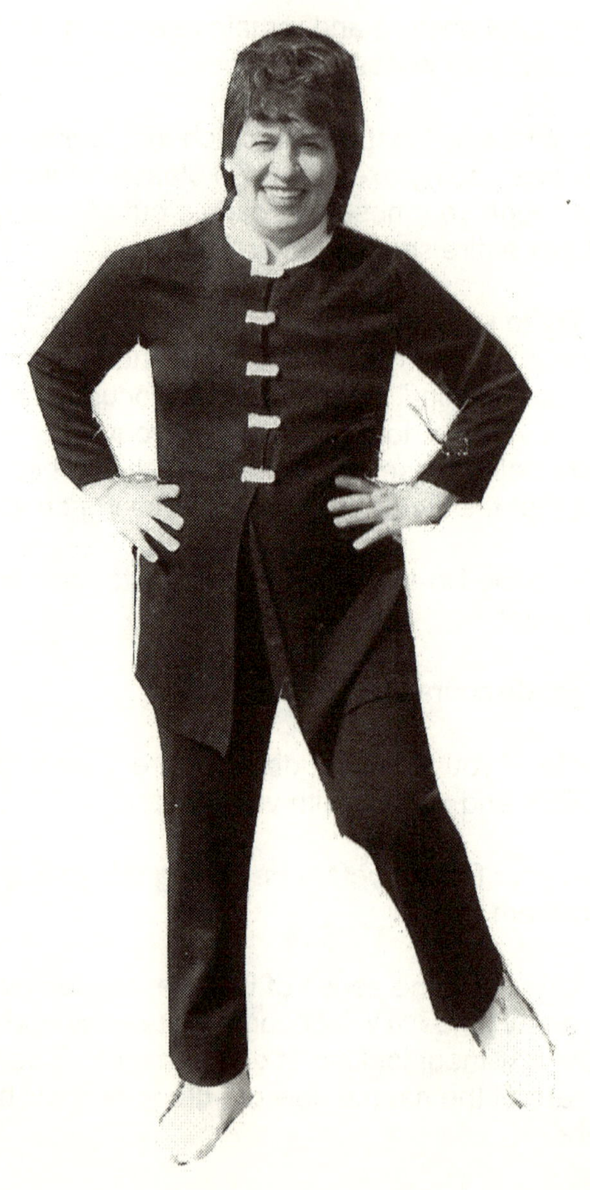

**To begin the series of DoIn exercises, you will first need to prepare your body.**

**How to prepare your body for the Do-In exercise routine:**

1. Stand up and begin to gently shake your body.

2. Shake your arms (Do 9xs)

3. Shake your hands (Do 9xs)

4. Lift your shoulders to your ears as your breathe in, then lower your shoulders as you breathe out. (Do 3 xs)

5. Then, lift you right leg a few inches off the floor and shake that leg. (Do 9 xs)

6. Then, shake your right foot. (Do 9 xs)

7. Then, lower the right leg and lift the left leg off the floor and shake that leg. (Do 9 xs)

8. Then, shake your left foot. (Do 9 xs)

9. When finished, sit in a chair or on a cushion on the floor until you are ready to continue on with the rest of the exercises.

Be sure that your spine is straight.

Enjoy the feeling of energy being released in your body; you are now ready to move on to the next lesson.

# Chapter Two

# Do~In Exercises

# Exercise #1-Top of Head

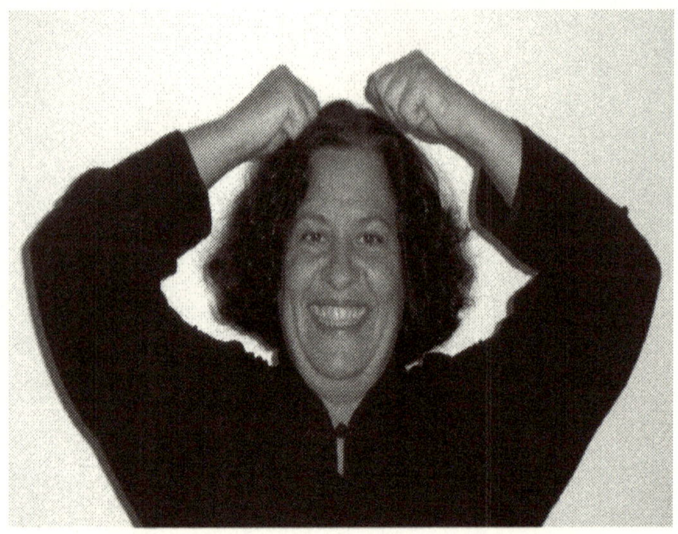

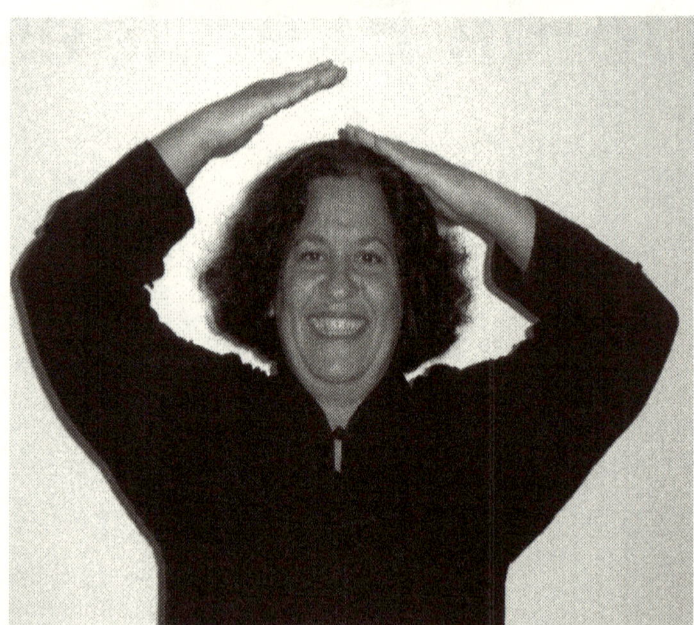

**To Do:**

Gently clench both hands, or leave them loosely open, and keep your wrists loose.

Start at the center top of your head and gently begin to alternate tapping your hands on your head.

Move your hands from the center to the sides of your head and from the sides of your head back to center.

Move your hands from the center to the back of your head and back to center again. Be sure to cover every inch of your head. Adjust the amount of pressure as needed.


**Benefits of Doing this Exercise**

Anterior Fontanel

(Helps with headaches, sinuses, hydrocephalus, aspirin poisoning, brain, spinal cord, central nervous system, controls cranial fluid)

Abdominal Cramps
Gas and Indigestion
Pyloric valve of stomach
Bloating/excess fluid
Coronary arteries
Intestines, Colon
Enlarged legs
Capillary system
Aids relaxation
Dizziness

**Exercise #2**

**Pulling Hair**

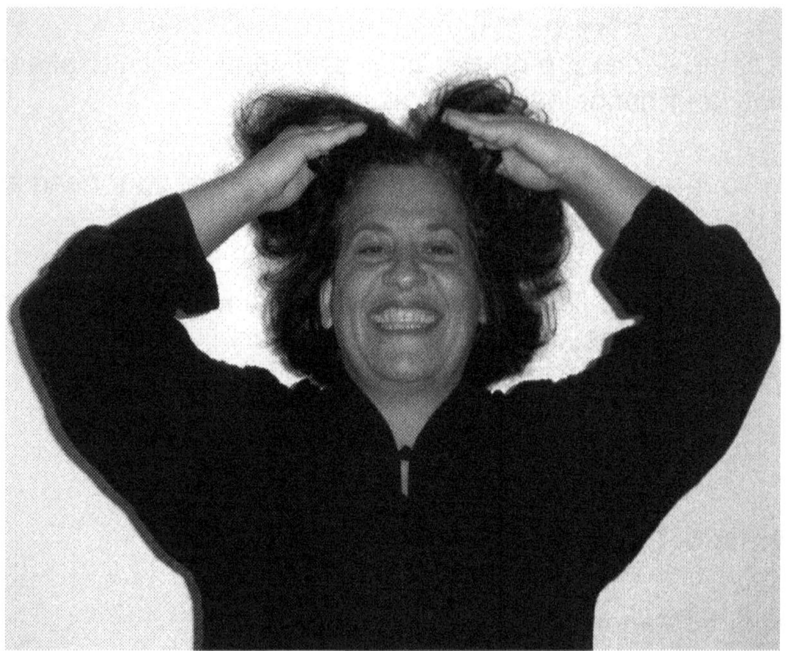

**To Do:**

Take your fingers and place them at the beginning of your
hairline. Now run your fingers through you hair and gently grasp
pieces of your hair and give them a gently tug.

Go through your whole this way, front to back, tugging on pieces
of your hair all over your head.

Do this for 1 minute.

**Benefits of doing this exercise:**

(This exercise will gently stimulate the meridians that runs cross the top and side of your head)

Bladder

Gall-Bladder

By doing this exercise, you will aid the following:

Asthma

Double Vision

Intestines/Stomach

Spinal Nerves

Aids relaxation

Capillary System

Brain

Abdomen

Excess fluid

Eyes

Heart

**Exercise #3**

**Back of the Head**

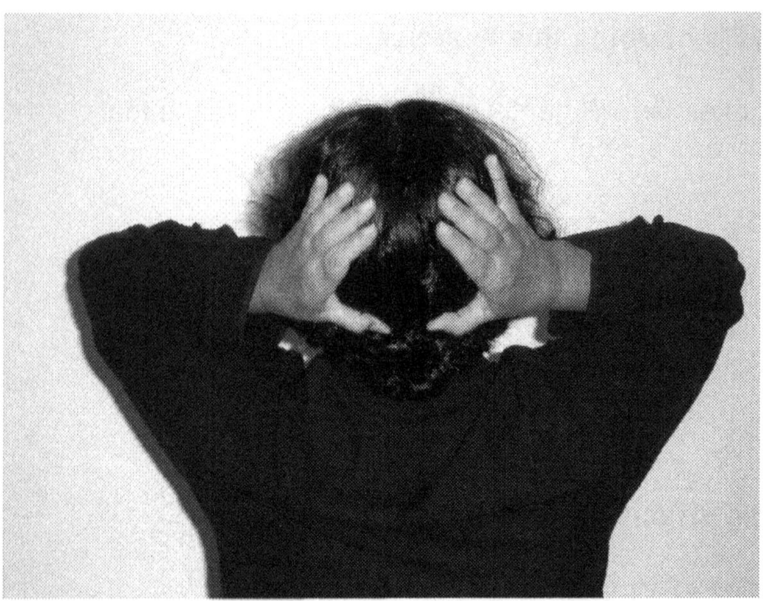

**To Do:**

Slightly lift your chin and place the thumbs of both of your hands on your earlobes. Your right thumb will be on your right earlobe and your left thumb will be on your left earlobe.

Now slide the thumbs back towards the center of your neck, one thumb width above the hairline of the neck. Your thumbs will fall into a depression on either side of the vertebra of your neck at the base of your skull.

GB20 is located in this depression. Use your thumbs to apply pressure to this point. Use medium to firm pressure and hold for at least 1 minute.

Breathe deeply and evenly while supporting your head with your fingers.

**Benefits of doing this Exercise**

Headaches

Colds

Neck stiffness

Neck pain

Tension Release

Stress Reducer

Helps to regulate the internal movement of energy

# Exercise #4

## Back of Neck

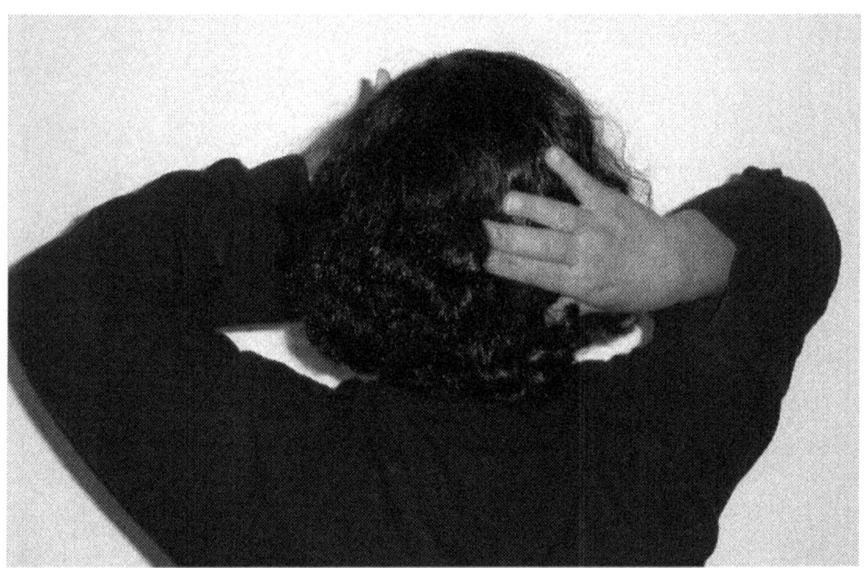

**To Do:**

Place your left hand on your forehead to support your head while you place your right hand on the back of your neck. Lift your chin up slightly.

Use the thumb of your right hand to gently stimulate the skull at the mid-base of your neck.

Vibrate your thumb gently as you apply pressure for about 1 minute and then release it.

Repeat this exercise for a total of three repetitions.

**Benefits of doing this exercise:**



Stroke

Pancreas

Gas

Indigestion

## Exercise #5

## Eyebrow

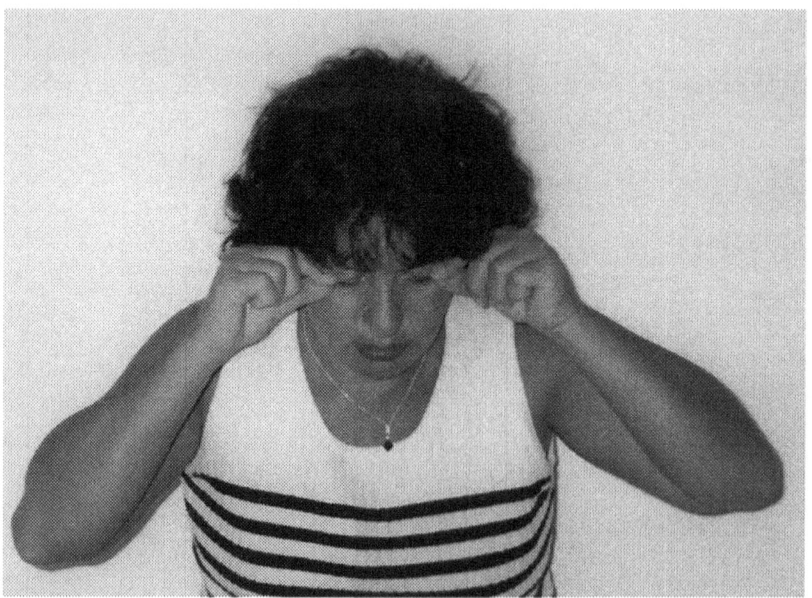

## To Do:

With your thumb and forefinger, 'pinch' your eyebrow starting from the inside of the eyebrow closest to your nose and working outward. Repeat for a total of three repetitions.

**Benefits of doing this exercise:**

Brain

Sinus

Eyes

Energy

Food poisoning

Gallbladder

Liver

Pleurisy

Sciatica

Eyestrain

Stomach

Stress

**Exercise #6**

**Nose**

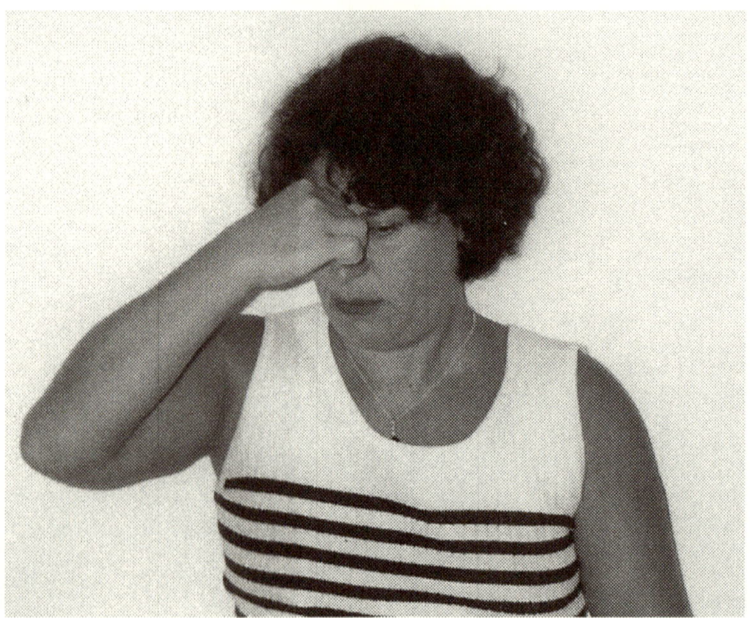

**To Do:**

With your thumb and forefinger, pinch the bridge of your nose
and hold for 1 minute. Release, and repeat for a total of three
repetitions.

Apply just enough pressure to feel the exercise but not too
much to injury yourself.

**Benefits of doing this exercise:**

Opens the eyes

Brightens the eyes

Clears the vision

Awakens tired eyes

Allergies

Sinuses

Sinus problems

Nasal problems

Nasal Congestion

Bronchi

Lungs

Benefits of doing this exercise:

# Exercise #7

## Under the eyes

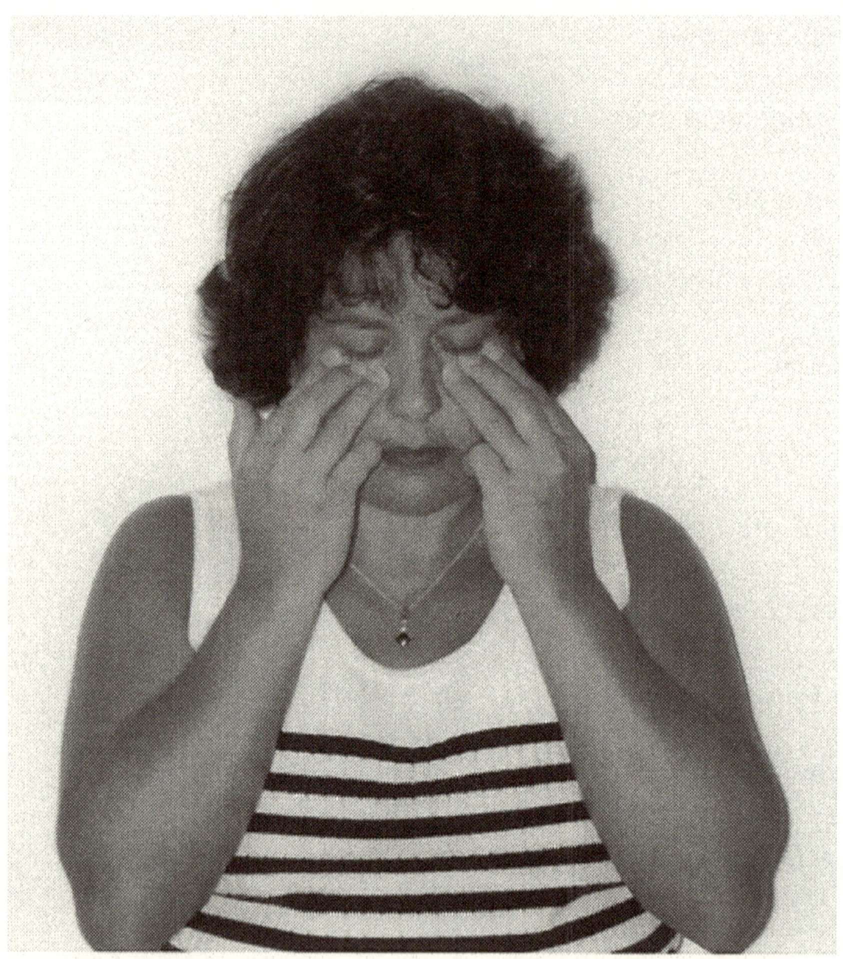

**To Do:**

Take the four fingers of both of your hands and place them on the top of your cheek bones located just under your eyes.

Apply pressure to this area and hold that pressure for 1 minute. Release that pressure and repeat again for a total of three repetitions.


**Benefits of doing this exercise:**

Aids in digestion

Stomach problems

Liver problems

Sinus problems

Nasal problems

Release mucus

Nasal stagnation and congestion

Anxiety

Allergies

# Exercise #8

## Under the Cheekbone

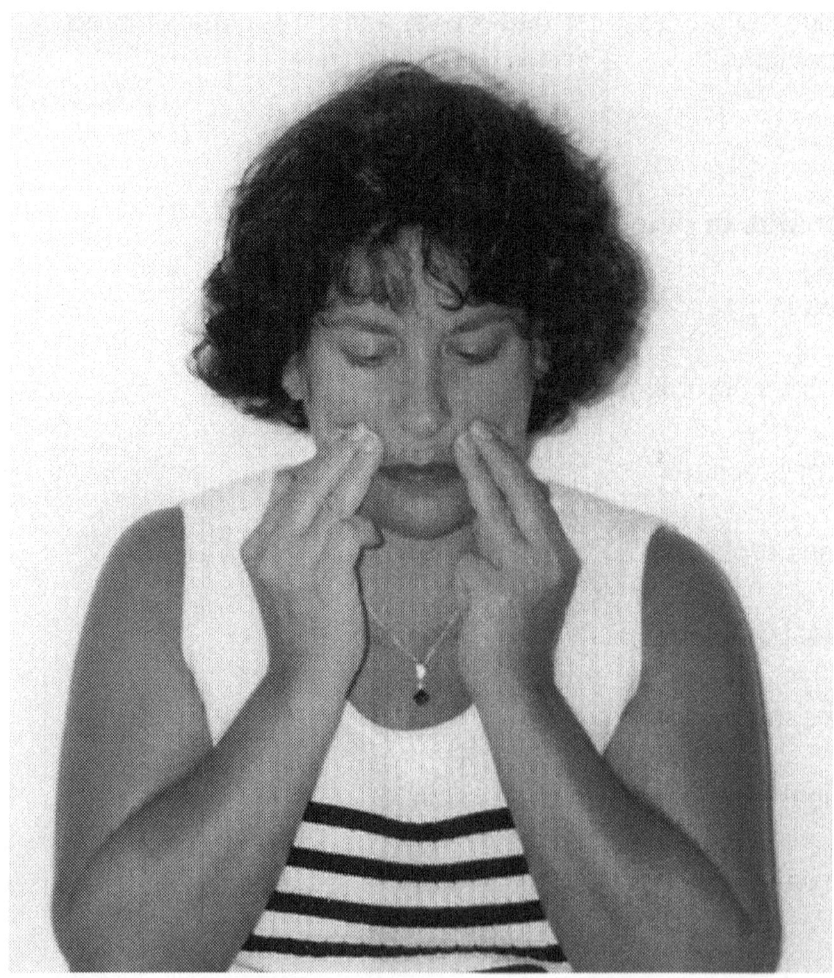

**To Do:**

Place the first three fingers of your hands on the area located just below your cheekbone and apply pressure there. Hold that pressure for 1 minute, release it, and repeat the exercise again for a total of three repetitions.

**Benefits of this exercise:**

Stomach problems

Digestion

Liver problems

# Exercise #9

## Chin

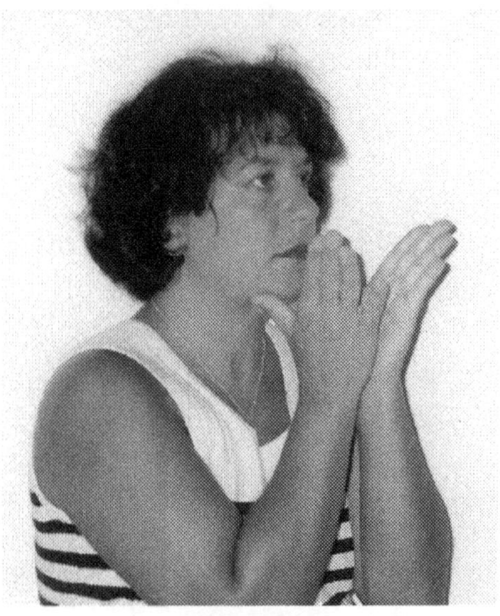

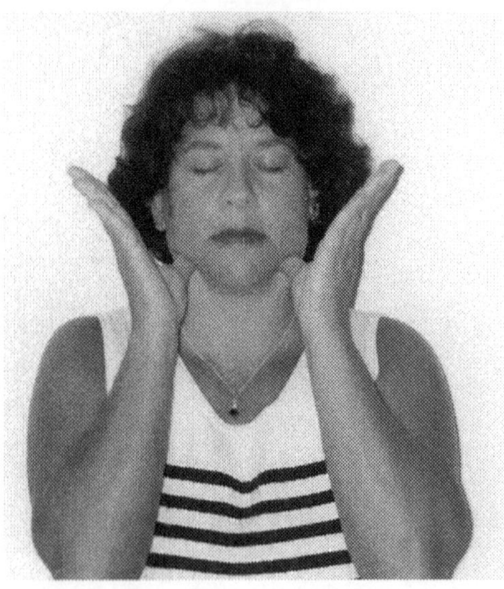

**To Do:**

Place both of your hands in front of your face with the thumbs of both hands resting under your chin. Your thumbs should be resting on the boney surface of your jaw line.

Now, while applying just the right amount of pressure, slide your thumbs down along your jaw line towards your ears.

Release and start over at the beginning of the jaw line in front of your face. Repeat this exercise for a total of three repetitions.

**Benefits of doing this exercise:**

Facial muscles and mumps

Ears, Eyes, Glaucoma

Saliva, Intestines, Amnesia

Lymph system

Aid relaxation

Aid TMJ and Jaw problems

Paralysis

Reproductive organ and Hysterectomies

Posterior Pituitary

# Exercise #10

## Sides of Face

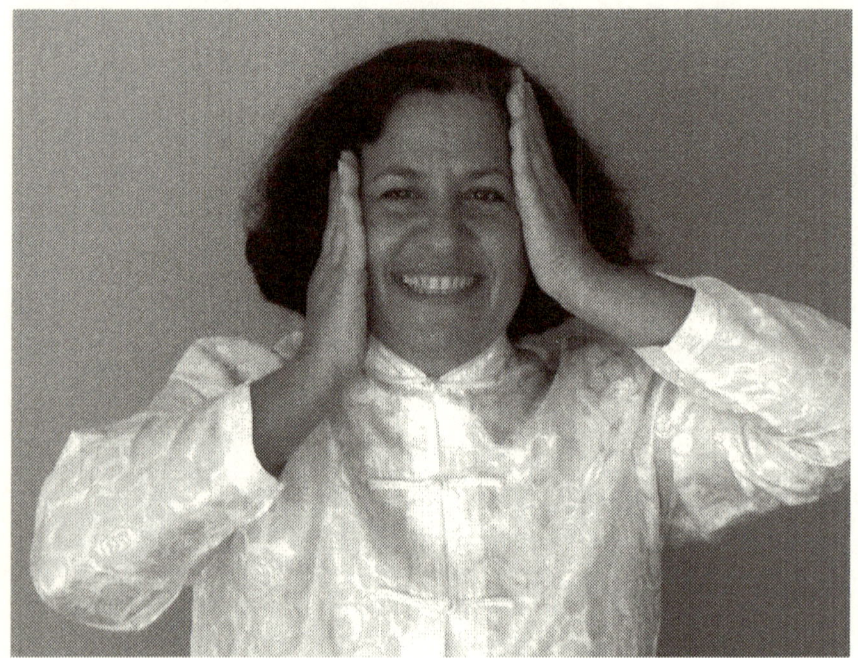

## To Do:

Place both of your open hands on your cheeks.

Begin to gently rub your cheeks in an up-and-down motion until the skin of your face becomes warm.

**Benefits of this exercise:**

Will help to stimulate the facial muscles

Relieves jaw pain and tension in the jaw muscles

TMJ

Lungs

Breathing

**Front of Face**

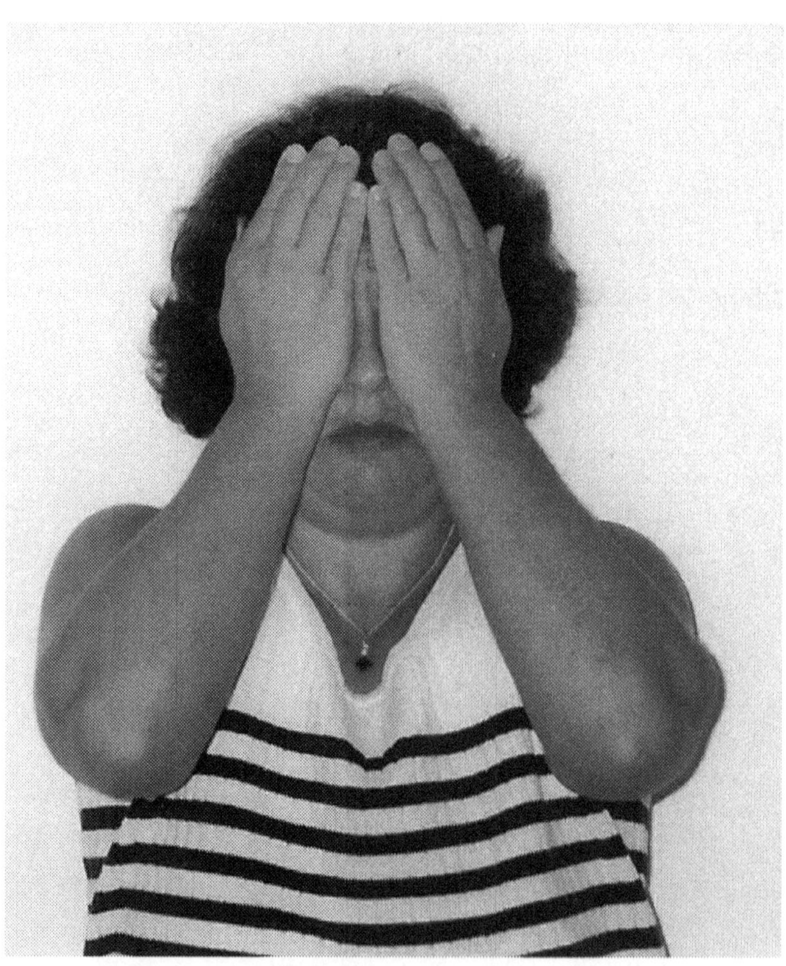

**To Do:**

Close your eyes and bring both of your hands to cover your face. Place the open palms of both of your hands over your eyes. Hold for 1 minute.

NOTE: Another way to accomplish this to rub both of your hands together first for 1 minute, then place the warm hands on your face for 1 minute.

This will bring both relaxation and circulation to your face and body. This exercise works great when you are under pressure and need a moment to yourself.

**Benefits of Doing this Exercise**

Brain

Sinus

Eyes and Eyestrain

Energy

Food poisoning

Gallbladder, Stomach

Liver, Stress

Pleurisy

Sciatica

# Ear Work

## Exercise #12

### Top of Ears

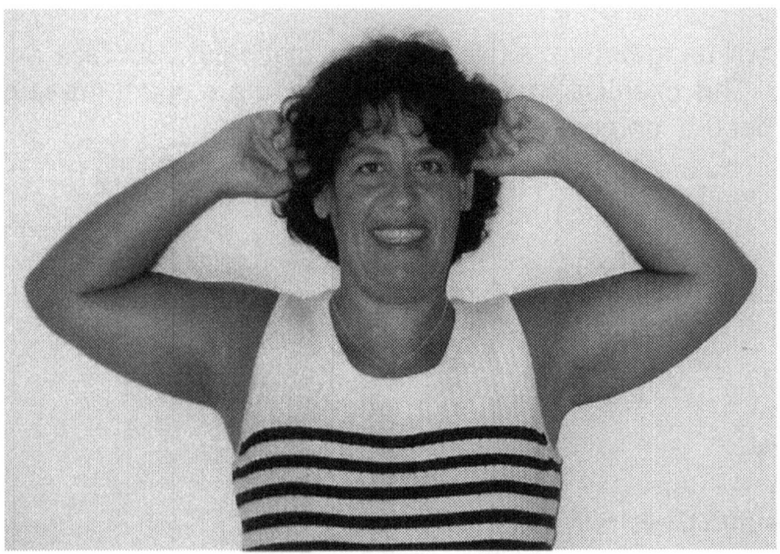

## To Do:

Grab the top of your ear with your thumb and forefinger and gently, yet vigorously, rub the entire area.

Do for one minute, rest, and repeat for a total of three repetitions.

**Benefits of doing this exercise:**

Toe

Heel

Ankle

Finger

Knee

Liver

Anus

Hip

Wrist

Blood Pressure

**Exercise #13**

**Backs of Ears**

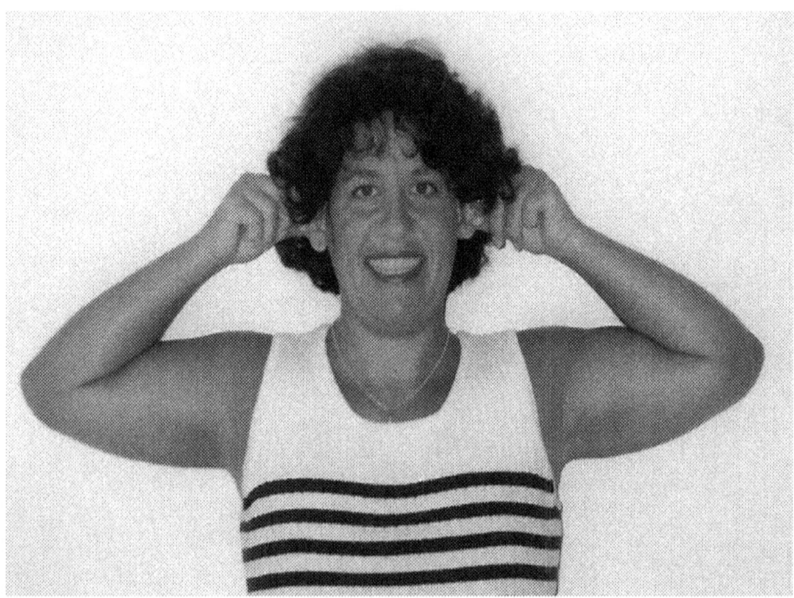

**To Do:**

Grab the back of your ear with your thumb and forefinger and begin to rub gently, yet vigorously, for one minute. Rest and repeat for a total of three repetitions.

**Benefits of doing this exercise:**

Elbow

Tonsil

Shoulder

Appendix

Lumbar Vertebra

Thoracic Vertebra

Cervical Vertebra

Thyroid gland

Clavicle

Neck

Mammary gland

Thorax

Liver

Abdomen

Chest

# Exercise #14

## Bottom of Ears (Earlobes)

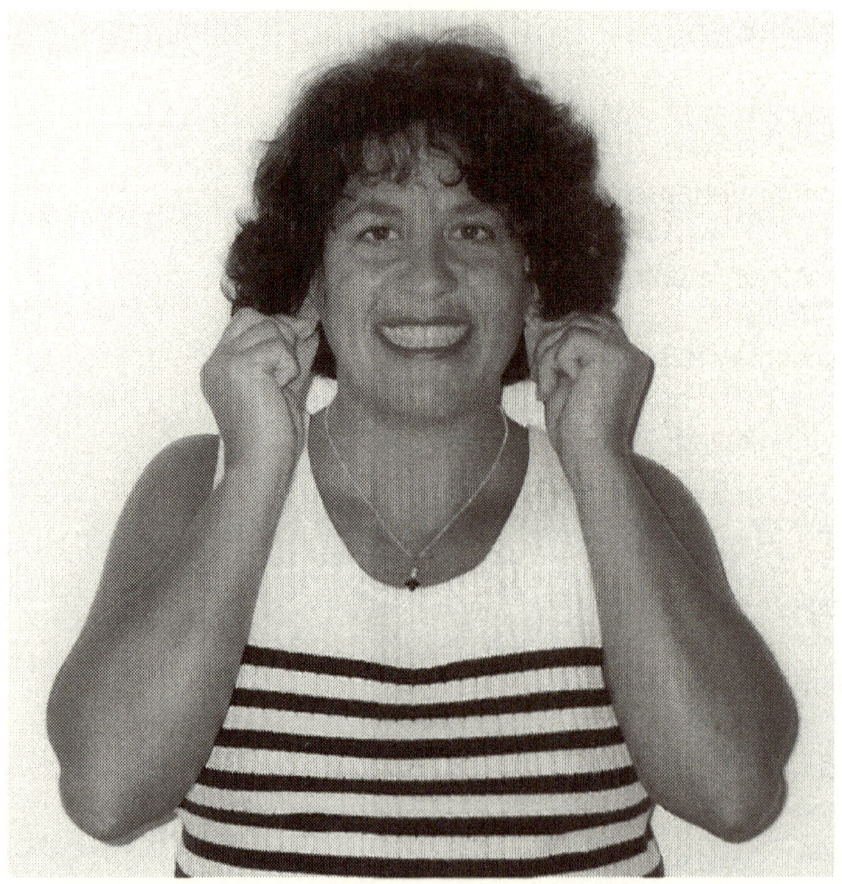

**To Do:**

Grab the lobe of your ear, the bottom part of your ear, between your thumb and forefinger.

Gently pull and stretch your ears up, out, and down.

Do this five times in each direction.

When finished, place the palms of your hands on your kidneys and hold them there for 3 to 5 minutes.

**Benefits of doing this exercise:**

This simple exercise is said to improve circulation and stimulate your kidneys.

## Exercise #15

## Shoulder

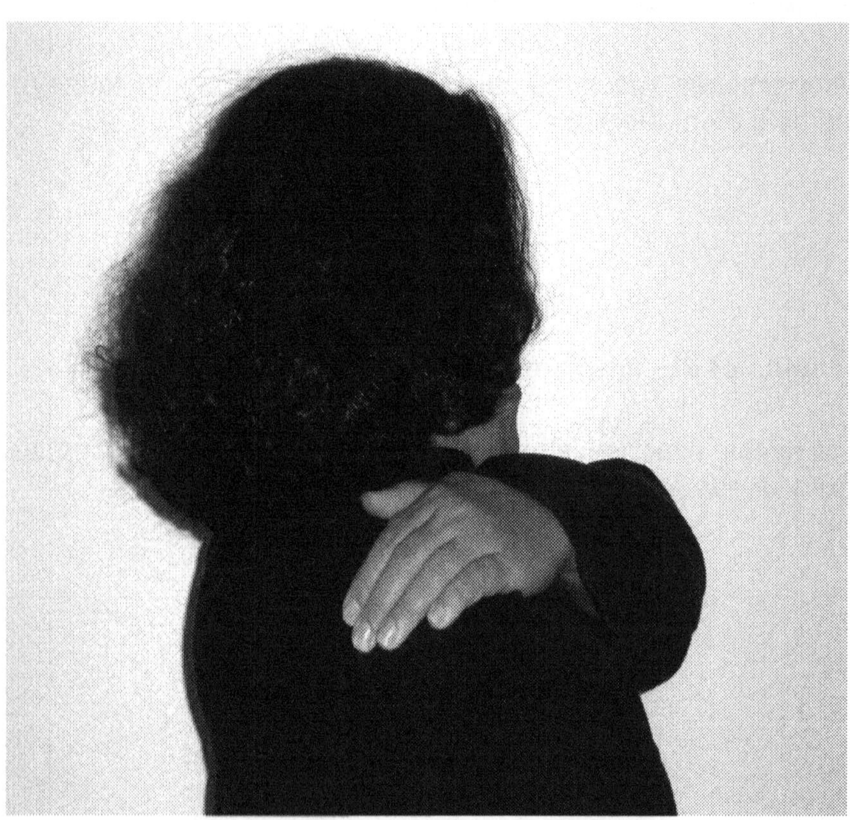

**To Do:**

Take your left hand and using either a fist, or an open palm, begin to gently tap your right shoulder for 1 minute. When finished, switch to your right hand and tap your left shoulder.

Repeat this exercise for a total of three repetitions which includes right shoulder/left shoulder, right shoulder/left shoulder, right shoulder/left shoulder.

Be sure to tap your hand as far back as you can reach over the shoulder blade. This is the location of the CB21 point otherwise known as The Shoulder Well.

**Benefits of doing this exercise:**

To relieve muscle tension

# Exercise #16

## Back of Arms

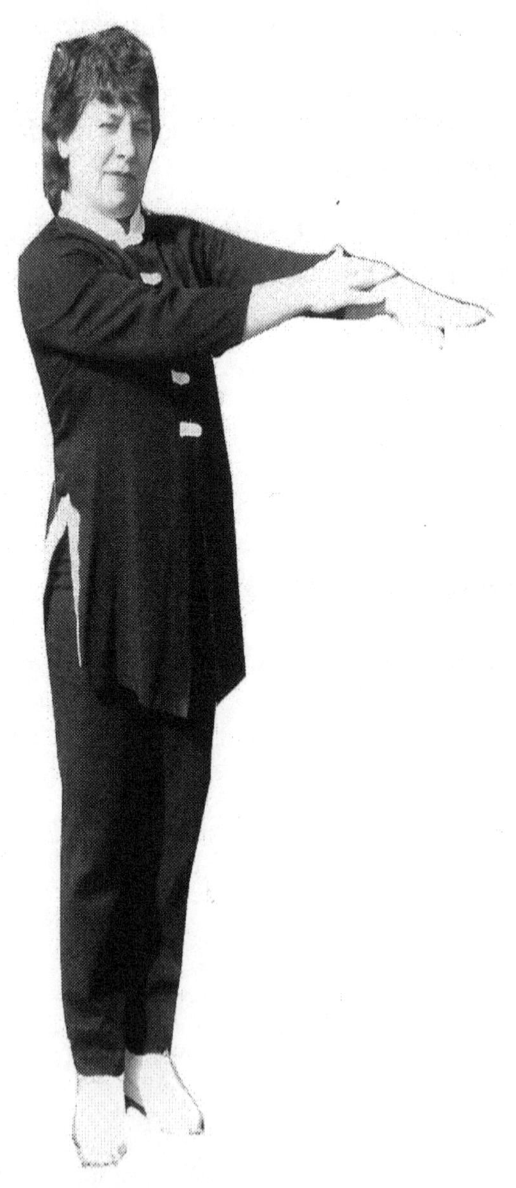

**To Do the Arm Exercises:**

Begin in a seated or standing position and extend your left arm out in front of you, with the palm of your left hand facing down.

Make your right hand into a fist, or leave it open if you prefer.

Begin at the top of your shoulder and gently start tapping down your arm down to your wrist and back up again to the top of your shoulder.

Do this for a total of three repetitions.

Then quickly follow with the next exercise before repeating the entire process on your right arm.

**Benefits of doing this exercise:**

Stimulates the energy flow of the lung

Heart Governor

Heart Meridians

Circulatory System

Respiratory System

Lungs

# Exercise #17

## Inside of Arms

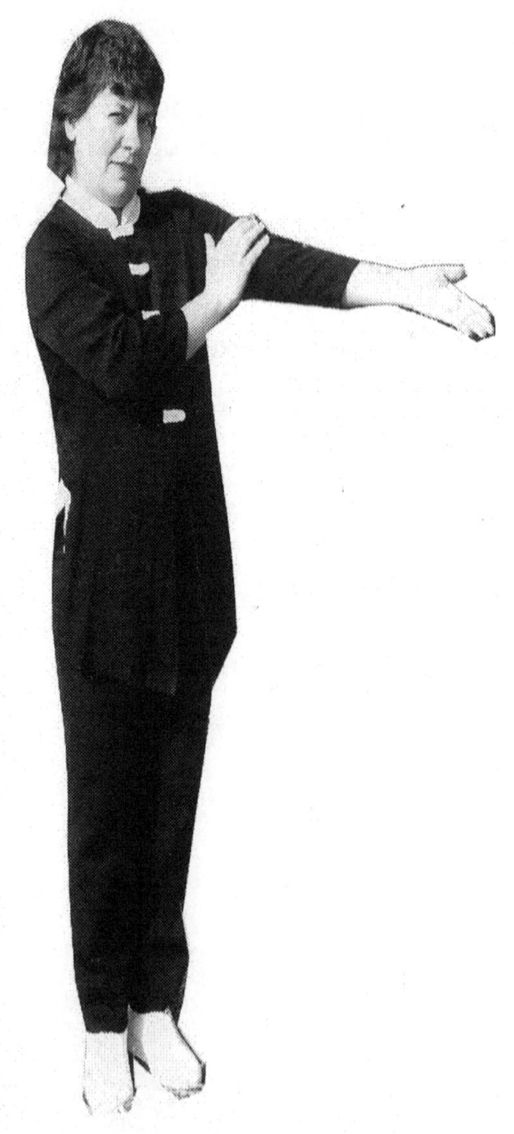

**To Do:**

Begin in a seated or standing position and extend your left arm out in front of you, with the palm of your left hand facing upward.

Make your right hand into a fist, or leave it open if you prefer.

Begin at the top of the inside of your arm (close to your armpit) and gently start tapping down your arm down to your wrist and back up again to your armpit.

Do this for a total of three repetitions.

When finished - extend your right arm out

Begin tapping your right arm with your left hand starting at the shoulder and moving on down to your wrist and back up again, then turn your right palm up and begin tapping the inside of your arm from your armpit down to your wrist and back up again.

Continue this tapping three times moving up and down the outside of your arm, then up and down the inside of your arm.

**Benefits of the exercise:**

Stimulates the energy flow

Large and Small Intestine

Triple Heater

Body Metabolism

## Chest and Back


## Exercise #18

## The Chest 1

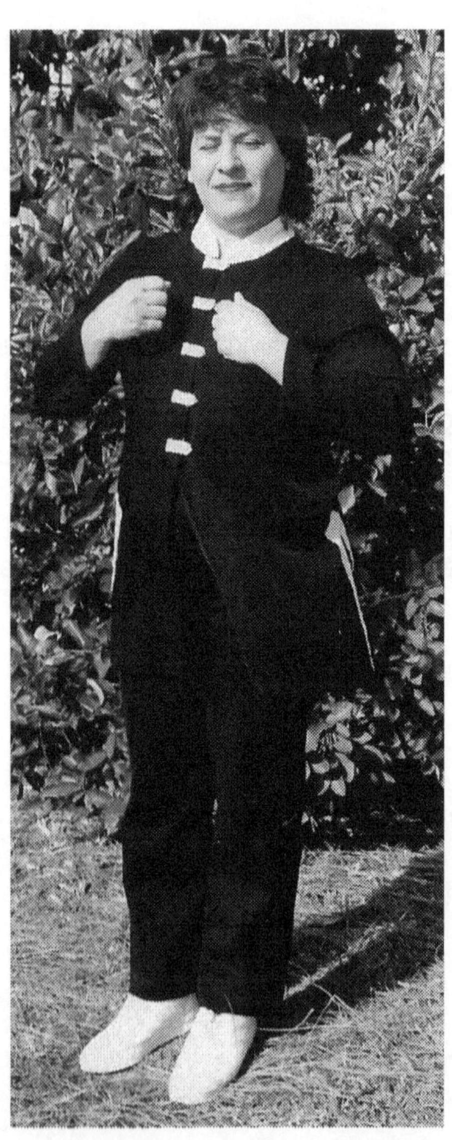

**To Do:**

Make your hands into two fists, or leave them open, and begin to gently tap all around your chest. Start from the center and move out to sides.

Do for 1 minute and rest. Repeat for a total of three repetitions.

**Benefits of Doing this Exercise**

Stimulates the lungs

Enhances and Strengthens the Respiratory System

Stomach

Pancreas

Spleen

Heart

Ears

Liver

Bloating and Indigestion

Lymph

Kidneys

Emotions

**Exercise #19**

**The Chest 2**

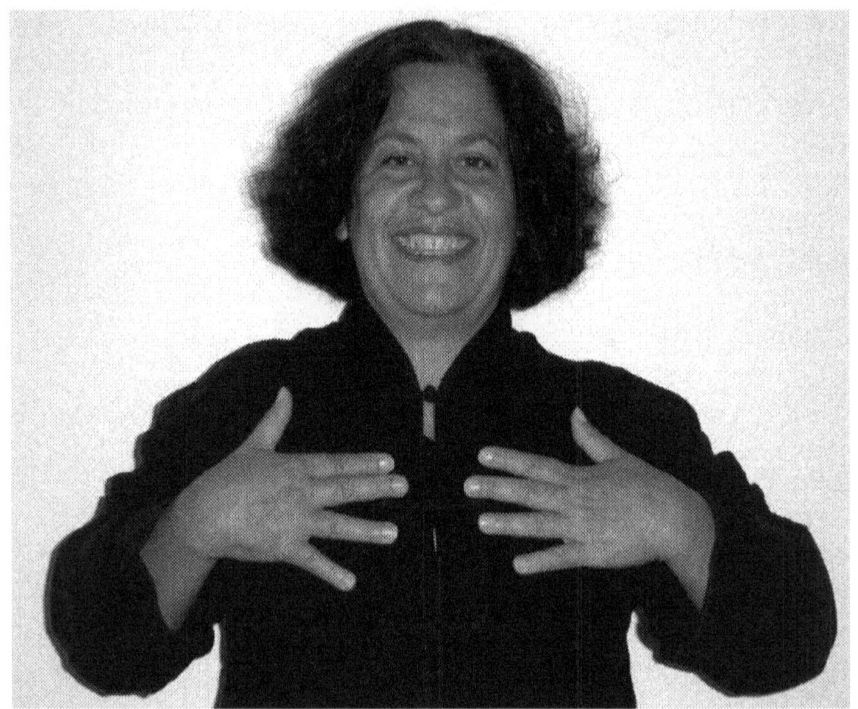

**To Do:**

Place your open fingers directly on the front center of your chest and add pressure while you pull your fingers across your chest towards the sides of your body. Continue to do this exercise for 1 minute, rest, and repeat again for a total of three repetitions.

You should feel nice warmth in your chest.

**Benefits of doing this exercise:**

Stimulates the lungs

Enhances and Strengthens the Respiratory System

Stomach

Pancreas

Spleen

Heart

Ears

Liver

Bloating

Indigestion

Lymph

Kidneys

Emotions

**Exercise #20**

**The Back**

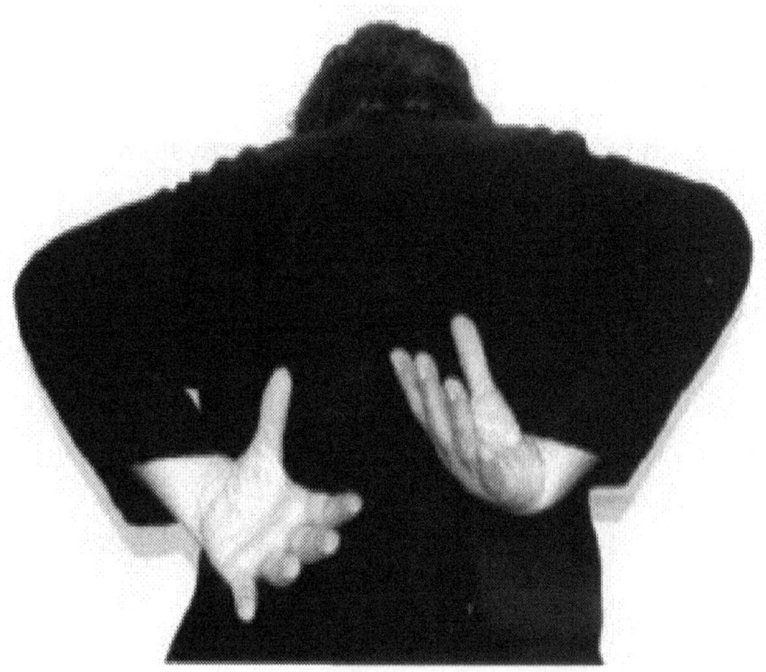

**To Do:**

Stand, or sit, with your feet shoulder width apart.

Bend your upper body slight forward and reach both of your hands behind you and gently tap your lower back with the backs of your hands.

Tap up and down your spine, over to your hips, and over the muscles of your buttocks.

Continue do this for at least one minute.

**Benefits of doing this exercise:**


Heart

Breathing

Pain

Releases Tension

Stimulates Digestive Organs

Stimulates Elimination Organs

Lungs

Flu

Fatigue

Shock

Stress

Leg Pain

Gall Bladder

Appendix

# Exercise #21

## The Spine

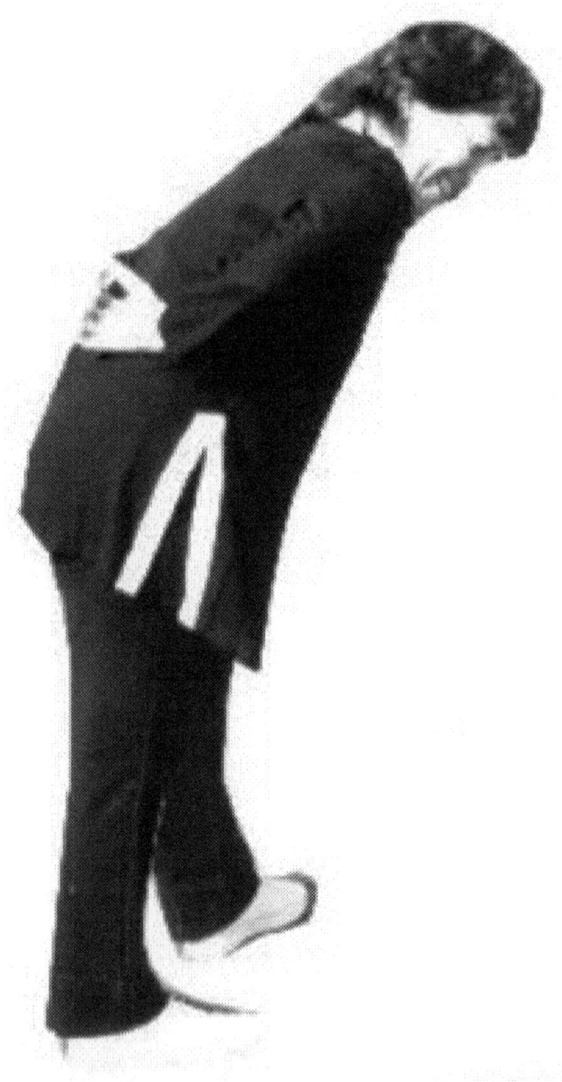

**To Do:**

Step your left foot forward and bend your torso slightly forward, supporting your body by placing your left hand on the front of the thigh of your left leg.

Use the back of your right hand and begin tapping across the sacrum bone at the base of your spine. Do this for 1 minute.

When finished, step your right foot forward and place your right hand on the front of the thigh of your right leg.

Use the back of your left hand and begin tapping across the sacrum bone at the base of your spine. Do this for 1 minute.


**Benefits of doing the exercise:**

This tapping will send energy vibrations up the spine to your brain.

Sinus decongestion

Leg pains

Tension in the hip

Activates the Nervous System

Tension in the abdomen

# Exercise #22

## The Kidneys

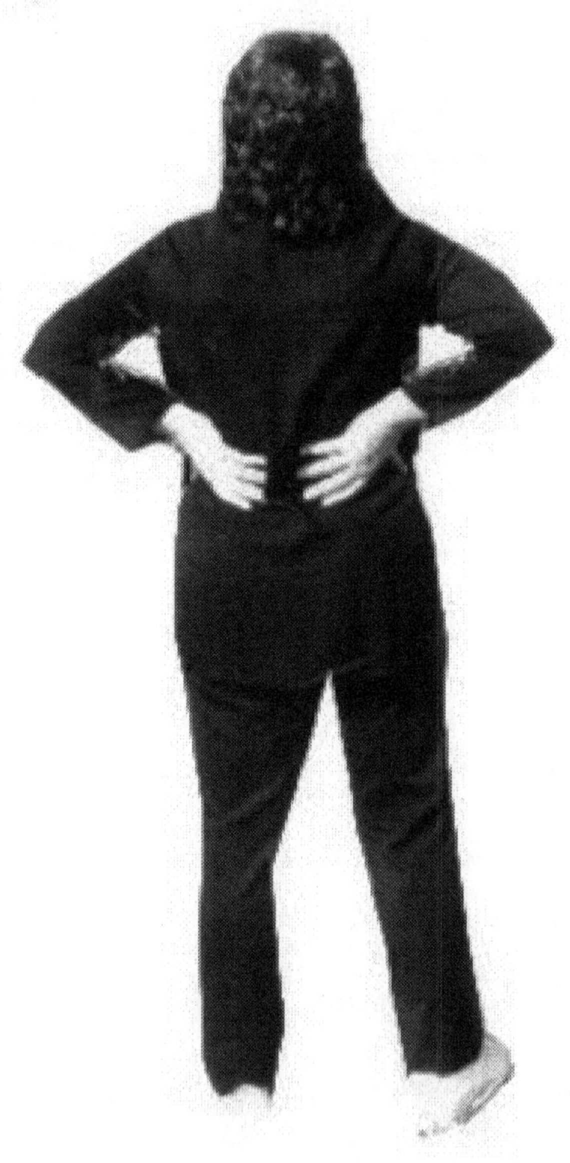

**To Do This Exercise:**

Stand with feet shoulder width apart

Place your hands on your back, below the rib cage and above your waist. (This is your Kidneys).

Start by rubbing this area slowly and gently with the palms of your hands.

Continue to rub until you feel warmth building up in this area.

**Benefits of doing this Exercise**

Your Kidneys have an important job to do in your body. They are responsible for the warming of your body and general vitality of your body.

The Kidneys are the storehouse for Qi, the body, and all the organs that Qi needs to thrive and be healthy. The health and vitality of each organ of your body depends upon the energy of the Kidneys. The Kidneys regulate the flow of water and filter about 360 gallons of blood a day.

# Exercise #23

## The Sides of the Body

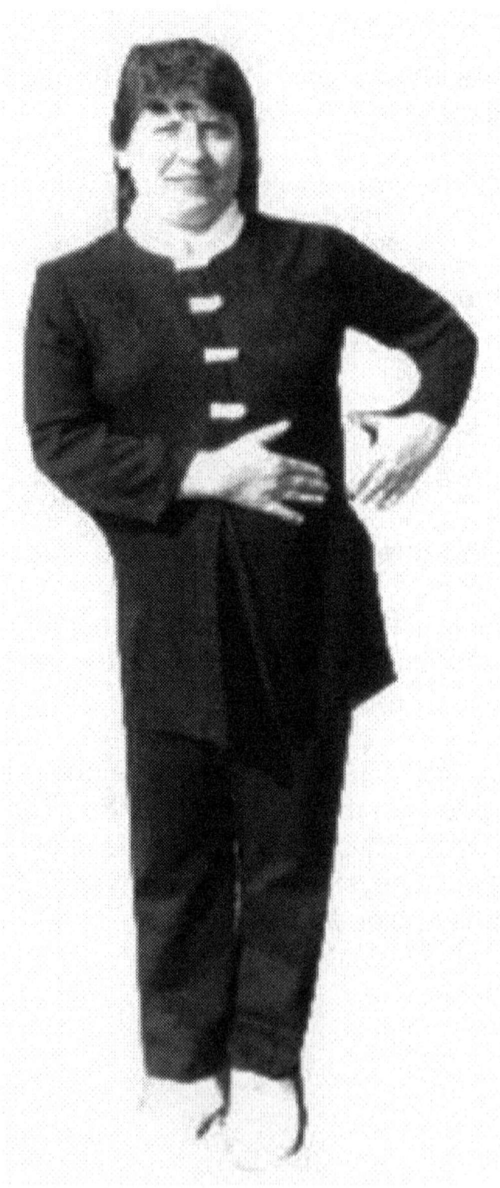

**To Do:**

Stand with your feet shoulder width apart and place your open hands on the left side of your body.

Begin to gently tap around your abdomen in a clockwise direction.

Go downward on your left side and upward on the right side. Do this for 1 minute on each side.


**Benefits of Doing this Exercise**


Aids the flow of circulation

Digestion

Constipation, Colon

Appendicitis, Spleen

Insulin

Gallstones, Lungs

Bile

Fast Heart

Flatulence and Abdominal Swelling

Pancreas

Legs


## Exercise #24

## The Front of the Legs

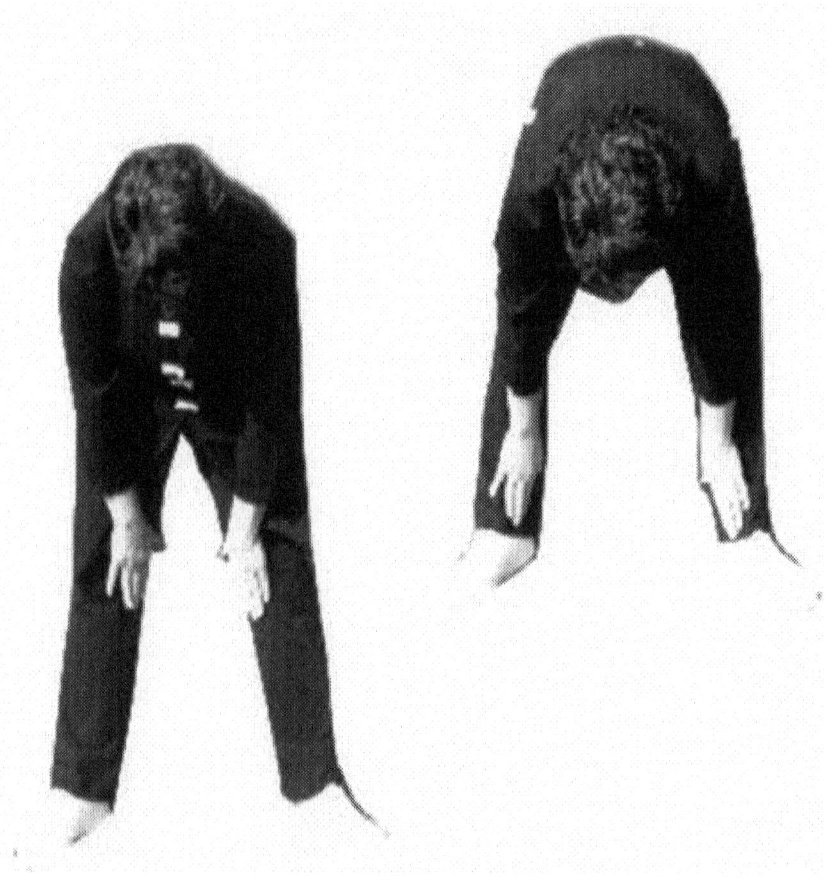

**To Do:**

Stand with feet shoulder width apart.

With open hands, begin to gently tap down the front of your legs to your feet, only if you reach that far, and back up the front of the leg again.

Do this for a total of three repetitions down and back up again.

**Benefits of Doing this Exercise**

Stomach

Hormones to the Heart

Dizziness

Bloating

Lung congestion

Diaphragm

Diabetes

Thyroid

# Exercise # 25

## Inside of Legs

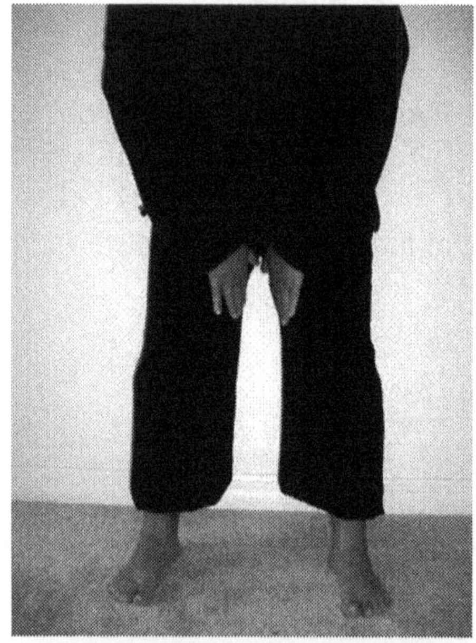

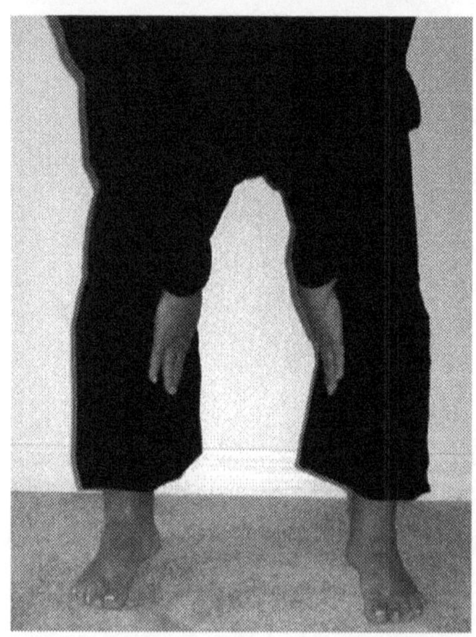

**To Do:**

Stand with your feet shoulder width apart

With open hands, begin tapping the inside of your legs beginning at your groin area and working down to your feet (if possible, if not, go down as far down the inside of your leg as you comfortably can go), and then tap back up the leg again.

Do this for a total of three repetitions.

**Benefits of Doing this Exercise:**

Lymph static

Mental confusion

Pituitary gland

Kidneys

Hormones

**Caution: Do NOT treat the lower leg during pregnancy**

# Exercise #26

## Sides of the Legs

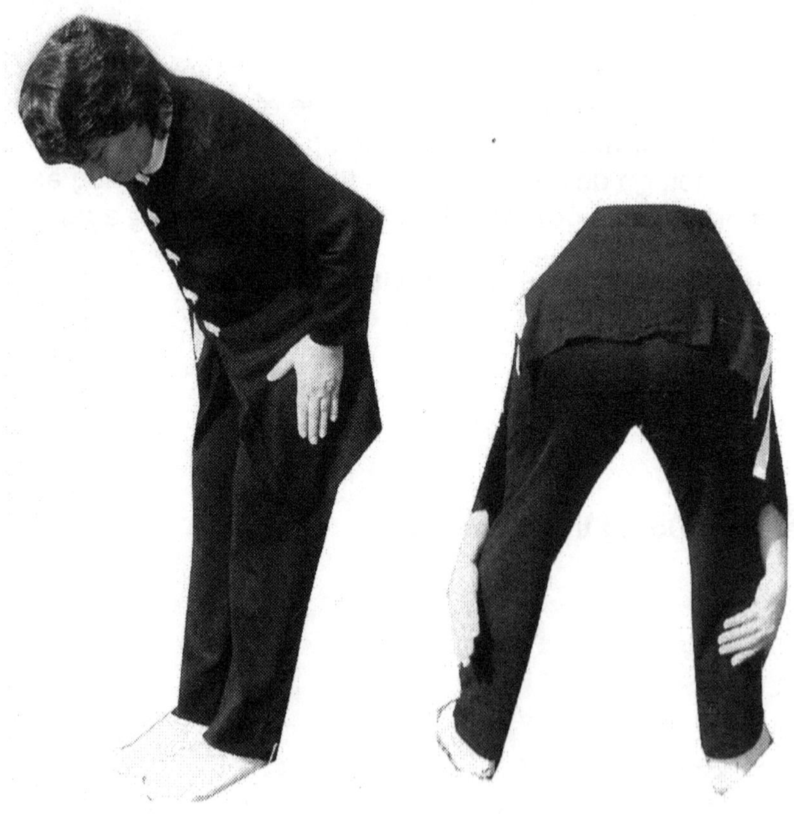

## To Do:

Stand with feet shoulder width apart and with open hands begin to gently tap down the outside sides of your legs to your feet, if you can reach that far, and back up the leg again.

Do for a total of three repetitions.

## Benefits of Doing this Exercise

Stomach

Abdominal lymph

Eyes

Feet

Muscles

Sprains

Strains

Diabetes

Obesity

Thyroid

Intestines

Heart

Tension

Colon

Hormones

Hip and Leg pain

**Exercise #27**

**Back of the Legs**

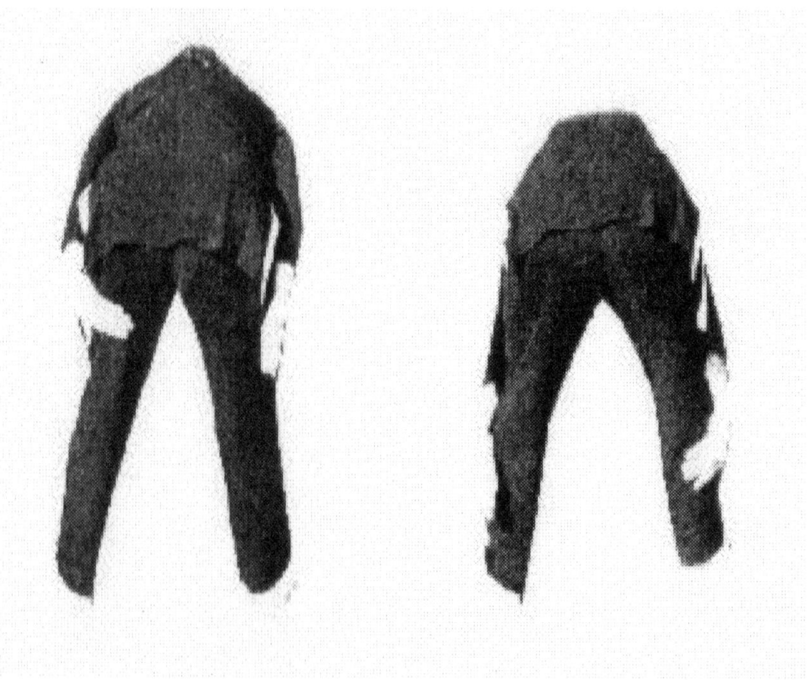

**To Do:**

Stand with your feet shoulder width apart

With open hands, begin tapping the back of your legs beginning at your buttocks and working down to your feet (if possible) and back up again.

Do this for a total of three repetitions.

**Benefits of doing this exercise:**

Bladder

Aching and Stiffness of the Legs

Joint pain in the legs and hips

Muscles

Colon

**Caution: Do NOT treat the lower leg during pregnancy**

## Exercise #28

### Spleen 6

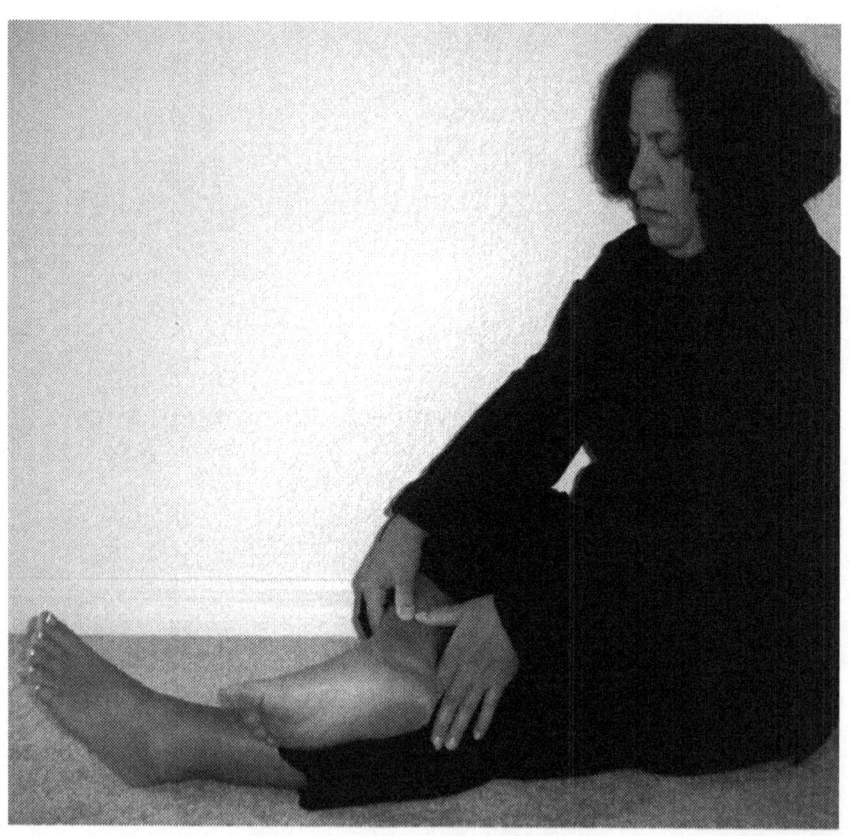

**To Do:**

Use your thumb and forefinger to massage the area located just under your ankle bone and to the back. The Spleen 6 point is located 4 fingers width up from the inside of the ankle bone.

Apply pressure on this point for 1 minute. Release and repeat this exercise for a total of three repetitions.

Adjust pressure as needed.

**Benefits of this exercise:**

Menstrual disorders

Spleen

Coccyx

**Exercise #29**

**Top of Foot**

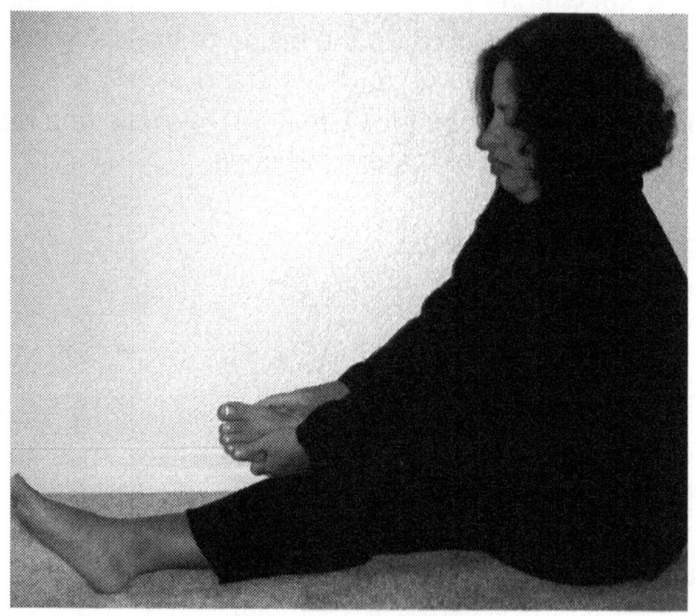

**To Do:**

Grasp your left foot with both of your hands and with your fingers underneath your foot. Your thumbs should be on the top of your left foot.

Use the thumbs of both of your hands to rub from the top of your foot downwards to the sides of the foot starting close to the ankle and working down towards the toes.

When you reach the toes, use your thumbs to rub between each metatarsal bone to your toes. (as shown in the picture below).

Do for 1 minute and then repeat on the other foot.

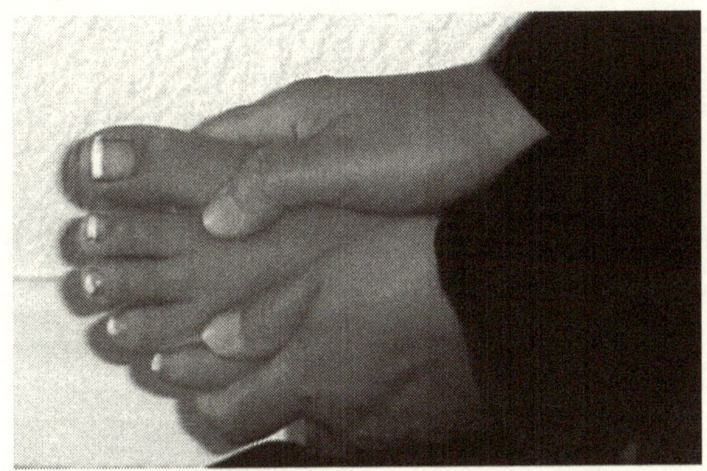

## Benefits of this Exercise

Breathing

Spleen

Pancreas

Ribs

Lungs

Breast

Neck

Thyroid

**Exercise #30**

**Sides of Foot**

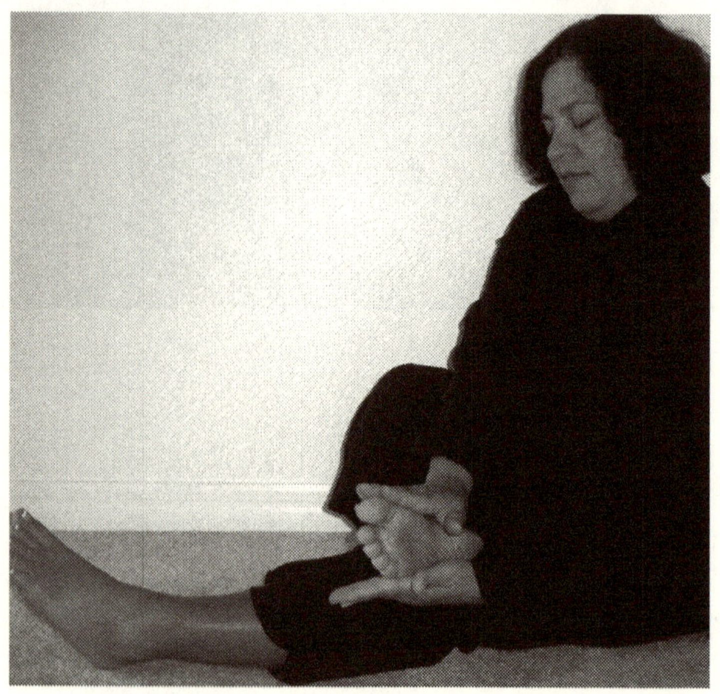

**To Do:**

Grasp your left foot with both of your hands and begin to gently rub the outside of your foot starting at the heel and ending at the toes, and back to the heel again.

Apply pressure as needed.

Do this exercise for 1 minute and then repeat on your other foot.

**Benefits of this exercise:**

Spine

Trachea

Bronchi

Sacral Vertebrae

Lumbar Vertebrae

Thoracic Vertebrae

Cervical Vertebrae

Coccyx Vertebrae and Coccyx Intestines

Constipation

Hipbones

Lungs

Mucus and Congestion

Feet

Constriction

Energy

**Exercise #31**

**Bottom of Feet**

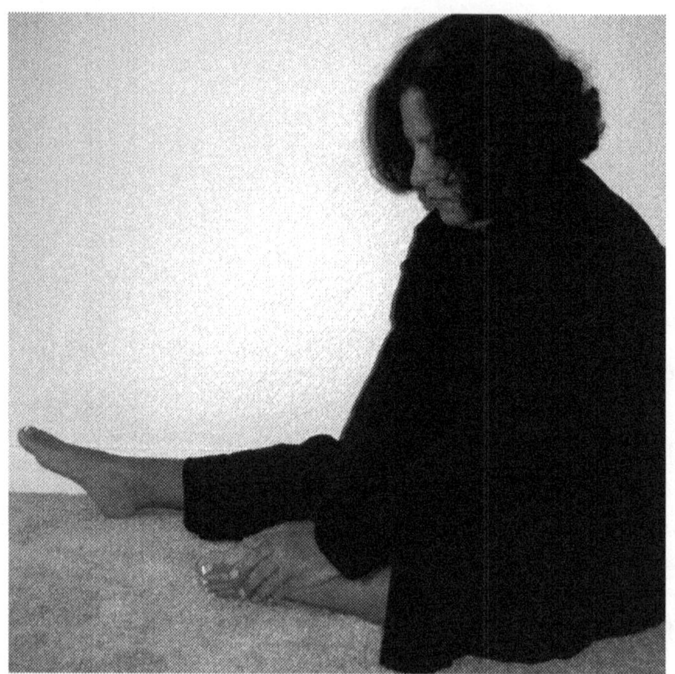

**To Do:**

Grasp your left foot in both of your hand.

Locate the center point at the bottom of your foot and begin to gently rub this entire area of your foot.

Do this exercise for 1 minute and repeat this exercise on your other foot.

**Benefits of this exercise:**

Gallbladder

Stomach

Thymus

Liver

Kidneys

Pancreas

Diaphragm

Lungs

Stagnation and Congestion

Kidneys

Circulation and Stimulate energy flow and Revitalization

Transverse and Ascending Colon

Small Intestine

Urethra tubes

Inflammation

# Exercise #32

## The Heel of your Foot

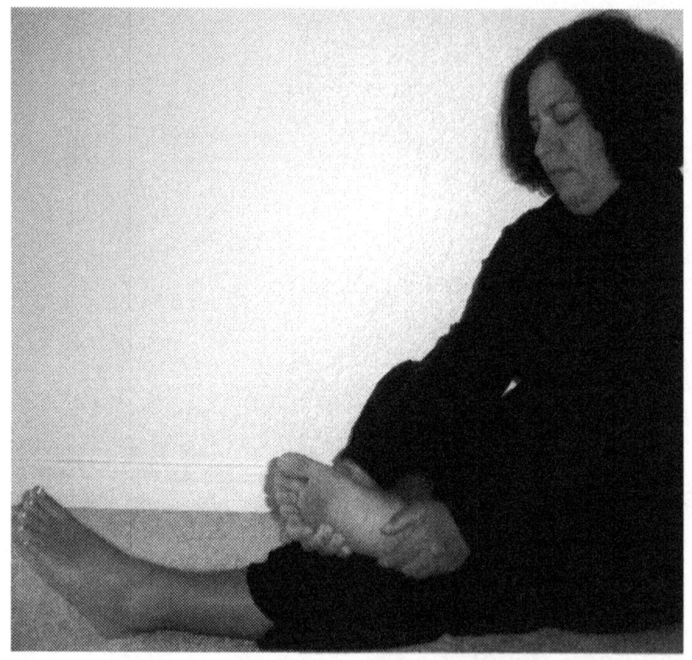

**To Do:**

Grasp your right foot in your right hand.

Make your left hand into a fist and begin to tap the sole of your right foot up and down the foot.

Do this for 1 minute and repeat the exercise on your other foot.

Follow this exercise with a total foot massage with open palms.

**Benefits of the exercise:**

Pelvis

Buttocks

Sciatic Nerve

Sigmoid Colon

Small Intestines

**Exercise #33**

**Ankle Rotations**

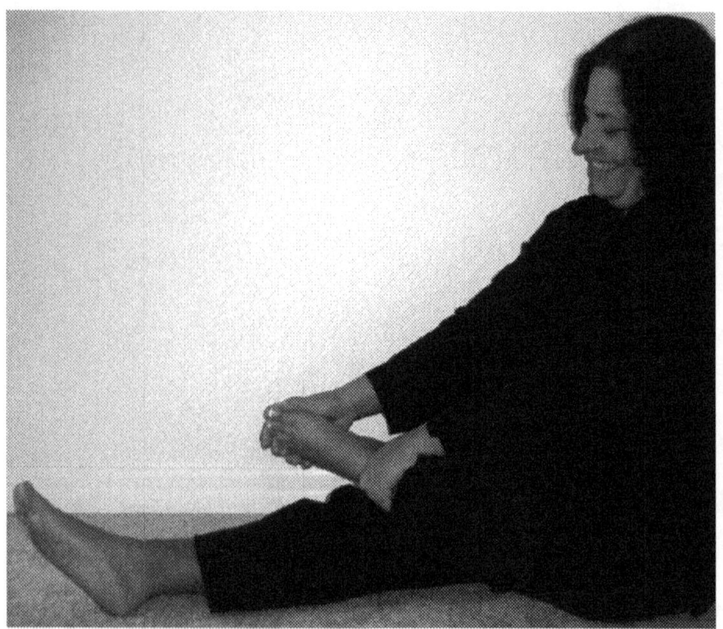

**To Do:**

Bring your left foot up in front of you and grasp the ankle of your left foot with your left hand.

Hold the top of your left foot with your right hand and gently guide your foot in a clockwise circular motion.

Do this for 1 minute, or for 45 rotations.

When finished, repeat this exercise on your right foot.

You should feel a warmth or heat in your ankle. Should you feel pain or discomfort, stop this exercise immediately and seek medical assistance. You should never work through pain.

**Benefits of the exercise:**

Blood circulation throughout the entire body

Sense of well being

Arthritis

Sore and tired feet

Sore and tired legs

## The Hands

## Exercise #34

### The Place of Anxiety

### Heart Governor 8

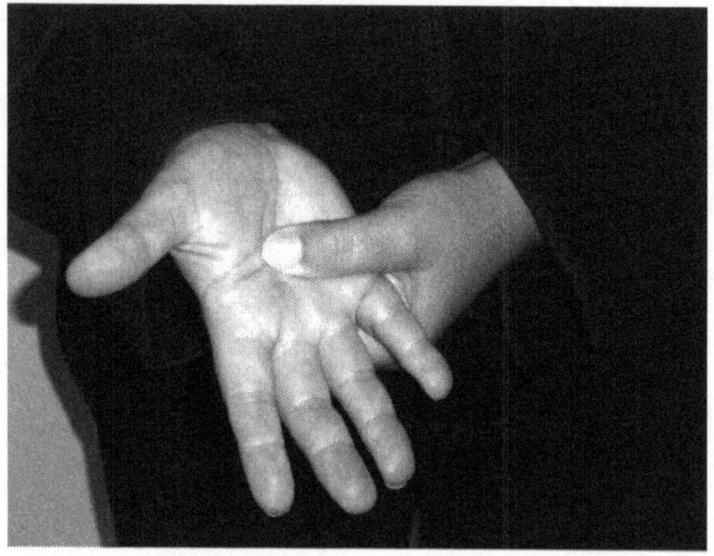

**To Do:**

Use the thumb of your right hand to gently massage the center of palm of your left hand. Adjust pressure as needed.

Do for 1 minute and repeat this exercise on your other hand.

**Benefits of doing this exercise:**

Use to relieve tension

Liver

Descending colon

Ascending Transverse colon

Stomach

Pancreas

Spleen

Bladder

Kidney

Urethra

**Exercise #35**

**The Fingers**

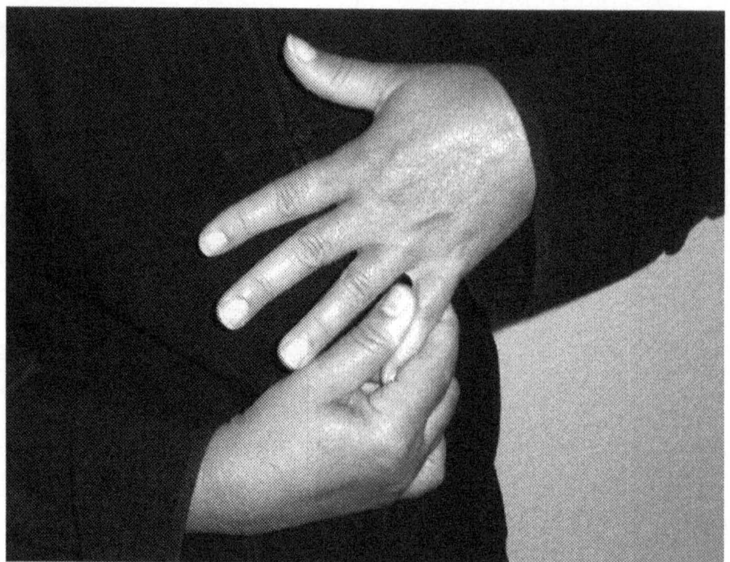

**To Do:**

Use the fingers of your right hand to take each of the fingers of your left hand and individually give each finger a little massage.

Start the massage at the base of the finger beginning with the thumb and working down the hand to the pinkie finger.

Be sure to gently rotate each of these digits while massaging them. Do this for 1 minute and repeat on the other hand.

**Benefits of this exercise:**

Sinuses

Eyes

Ears

Neck

Thyroid

Brain

Pituitary Gland

Pineal Gland

## Exercise #36

## LI4

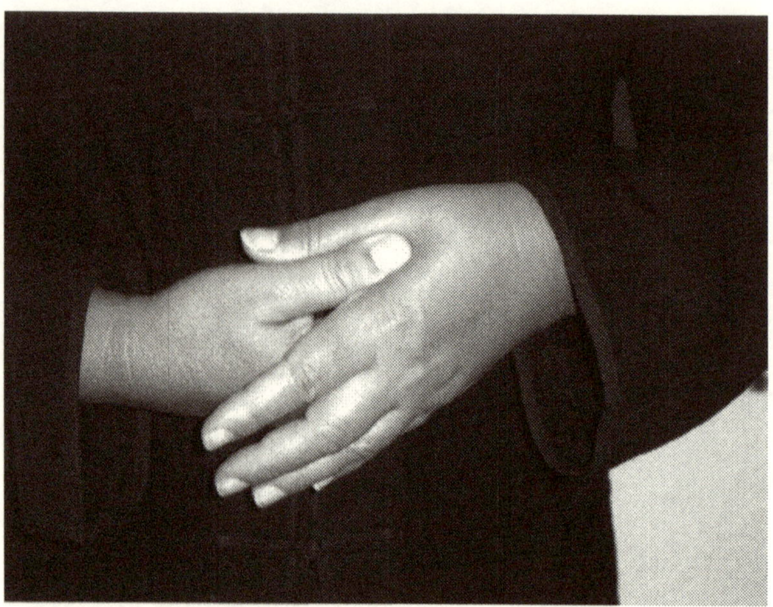

## To Do:

Take the thumb and forefinger of your right hand and apply
pressure to the area of your left hand between the thumb and
index fingers. This is the area of your hand that forms a V.

Do this for 1 minute and then repeat this exercise on your other
hand.

**Benefits of this exercise:**

This area is sometimes called the 'Pain Point' and can be used whenever there is pain in the body.

Relieves headaches

Constipation

Diarrhea

Pain

Stimulates labor

**Caution: Do NOT this point during pregnancy.**

**The Completion**

Below is the list of exercises that you have learned through this course.

You are now ready to put them all together.

Starting with the top and your head, you begin by gently tapping the top of your head, work through pulling your hair, tug at your ears, hold your mouth points, work your eyebrow points, rub your cheeks, place hands of face, then work your neck, head, chest, back, front of legs, inside of legs, back of legs, feet, and finally the hands and fingers.

If you skip an exercise or do them out of order, do not worry. It does not matter if you prefer a different way to do these exercises. Do what comes naturally for you and your body. All that is important is that you DO the exercises.

After you have completed this set of exercises, remember to sit comfortably and quietly for a few minutes and enjoy the vitality of your body.

These exercises are recommended for the morning, or you can use them throughout the day when needed.

Do NOT do these exercises before bedtime.

Remember to breathe deeply and normally.

This set of exercises should only take you a few minutes do to, so allow yourself this time to nurture yourself. You deserve it!

Enjoy!

# Chapter Three

# Additional Exercises

# Abdominal Massage

## Exercise #37

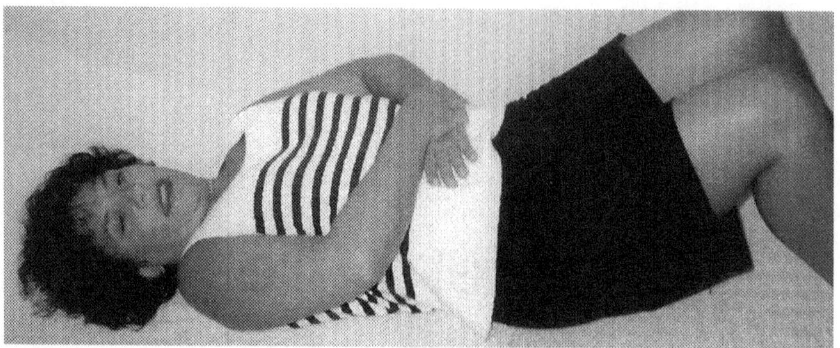

**To Do:**

While lying on your back with your knees bent, relax your stomach muscles.

With your right hand, grab the wrist of your left hand. With the four fingertips of your left hand, push slowly and deeply first on the right side of the abdomen from bottom to top, then on the left side of the abdomen from bottom to top.

Exhale each time that you press down and lift your hand up quickly.

Now, do the upper part of the abdomen from right to left, the right side from top to bottom, the lower abdomen from left to right, and the center from top to bottom.

Repeat the cycle for three repetitions.

Then, holding your right hand on top of your left hand, massage the navel area with the palm of your left hand in a circular motion.



**Benefits of doing this exercise:**

To relax abdominal muscles

To stimulate the organs in that area

To aid digestion

Relieve constipation

# Exercise#38

## Alternate Nostril Breathing

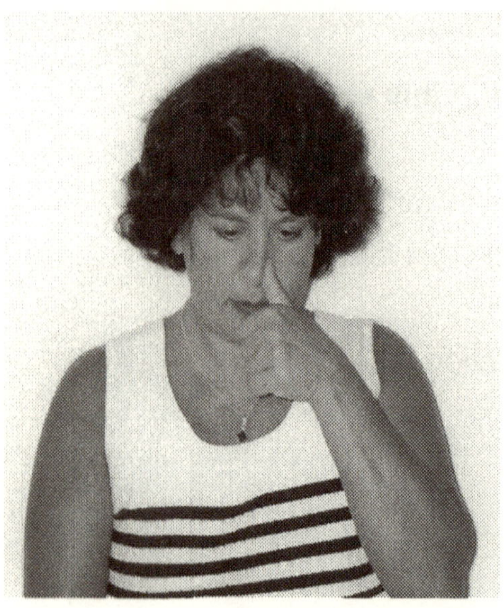

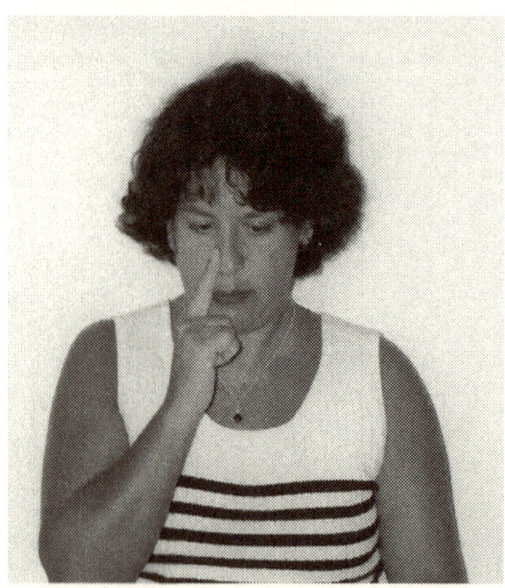

**To Do:**

With the thumb or index finger of your left hand, close off the left side of your nostril and only breathe through your right nostril.

Breathe in slowly and deeply and exhale slowly and mindfully. Do this for three repetitions and then breathe normally.

When finished, take the thumb or index finger of your right hand and close off the right side of your nostril. Breathe only through your left nostril.

Breathe in slowly and deeply and exhale slowly and mindfully. Do this for three repetitions and then breathe normally again.


**Benefits of doing this exercise:**

Promotes relaxation

Releases tension and stress

Headaches

Meditation

Balances the right and left hemispheres of the brain

Releases anxiety

Increases oxygen intake

# Chapter Four

## Microcosmic Orbit

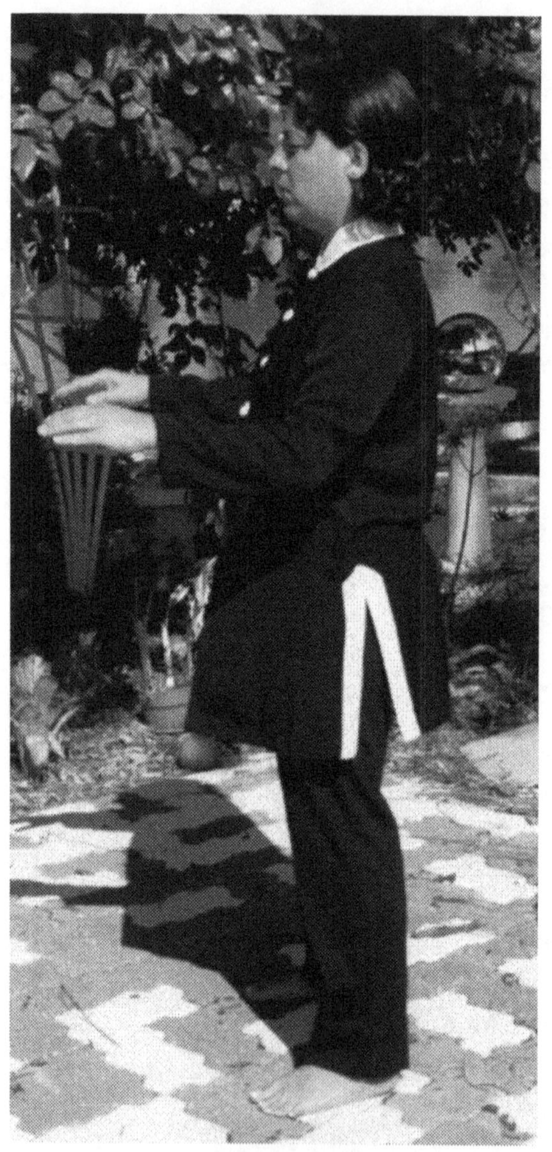

## The Six Posture Cues for performing the Microcosmic Orbit


1. Stand Erect, with the top of your head reaching upward. Your chin should be drawn slightly in.

2. Keep your head straight with your eyes softly focused and gazing downward at about a 45 degree angle.

3. Lower and relax your shoulders and allow your arms to bend at your sides with your hands reaching out in front of you at a right angle. Spread your fingers slightly and relax them.

4. Relax your abdomen so that you can take breaths without constriction.

5. Relax your hips and buttocks. Keep your knees soft and unlocked.

6. Stand with your feet shoulder width apart and parallel to each other. Your weight should be evenly distributed between your left and right feet.


NOTE: Although not necessary, performing the Microcosmic Orbit after completing the series of Doln exercises can be a very healing and powerful experience. I highly recommend it.

**TO DO:**

Put your tongue on the roof of your mouth and take a long, slow deep breath in through your nose. Take that breath down the front of your body to the Hui-Yin point which is located at the bottom of your torso between the scrotum and the anus (or posterior vulva and anus in women).

As you exhale, force that exhalation up your back and over your head to your nose. Inhale again bringing that breath down the front of your body and exhale bringing that exhalation up the back of your body and over your head to your nose.

You will be performing a complete circle of inhalation and exhalation with the breath. This is very powerful. Taoists believe that when these two main energy systems circuits, the Conception and Governing Channels are in sync, that energy will flow strongly and smoothly.

When out of sync, energy will become plugged up or 'leak out', especially at the joints.

It takes 100 days of daily practice to store up enough energy to circulate it throughout the channels of your body. But it is well worth it.

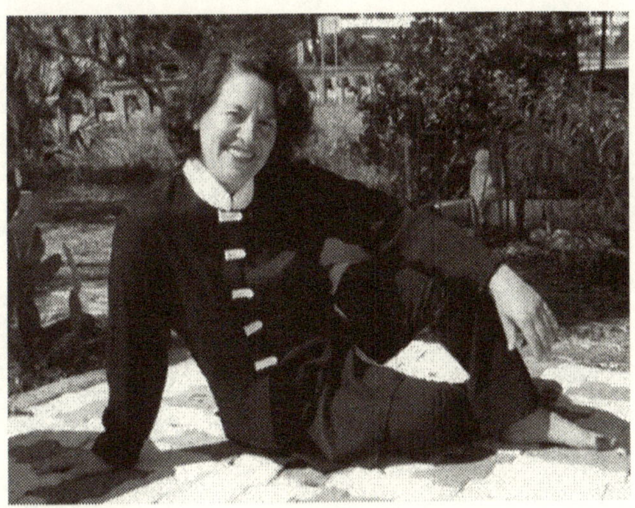

Francine Milford has had a very long career in the Fitness Industry. Working for more than twenty years in a variety of sports and exercise related classes, she is also an avid walker and enjoys reading a book audio tape while bicycling around the neighborhood.

She has achieved certifications through the YMCA S.A.F.E. Aerobic Program, AEA Aquatics Exercise Association, ESA Exercise Safety Association, and AFAA Aerobics Fitness Association.

Francine has also received the Tai Chi for Arthritis Certification having studied under Dr. Paul Lam, as well as, 180 hours of professional training in Tai Kwan Do.

She has taught such classes as Kick Boxing, Bench Stepping, Low Impact Aerobics, High Impact Aerobics, Basic Floor and Senior Aerobics and all types of Water Aerobic classes.

As a personal trainer and fitness specialist, Francine has been hired to lead classes and workshops at offices, condo organizations, clubs and private groups.


Having spent the last ten years working with the senior population, Francine has developed exercises that are both safe and effective for those with physical limitations.

# References


American College of Sport Medicine, Guidelines for Graded Exercise Testing and Exercise Prescription. Philadelphia: Lea and Febiger, 1995.

Beasley, Bob L., et al. "Metabolic and Heart Rate Responses to Aquatic Exercise," Research Council Proceedings-Southern District, American Alliance of Health, Physical Education, Recreation and Dance, 1987.

Chen, Pin. Modern Chinese Ear Acupuncture. Paradigm Publications, 2004.

Hoeger, W.W.K. Principles and Labs for Physical Fitness and Wellness. Englewood, CO: Morton Publishing, 1999.

Phil, Mark Evans B, FNIMH. The Guide to Natural Therapies, Choosing and using natural methods for physical and mental well-being. Anness Publishing Limited. 1996.

Practical Ear-Needling Therapy, Medicine & Health Publishing, Co., Published in Hong Kong. April 2002.

www.ingramcontent.com/pod-product-compliance
Lightning Source LLC
Chambersburg PA
CBHW031143250726

48655CB00002B/816